Molly Top's
Teen Guide to
Love, Sex,
and No Regrets

MOLLY TOP'S
TEEN GUIDE TO
LOVE, SEX, and NO REGRETS ♥

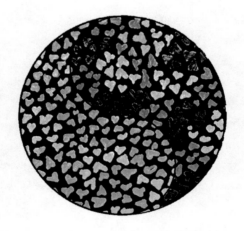

♥ Changing the World One Kiss at a Time

Elizabeth L. Clark

Copyright © 2012 Elizabeth L. Clark
Lightning Source Edition

ISBN 978-0-9836203-1-0 (paperback)
ISBN 978-0-9836203-0-3 (ebook)

Cover design by Elizabeth L. Clark and Shelly L. Francis
Book design by Shelly L. Francis
Thanks to dafont.com for the fun title set in Classroom Boredom courtesy of John Laubach and Mia's Scribblings by Amelia McVinnie.

While we hope the information in *Molly Top's Teen Guide to Love, Sex, and No Regrets* will help you make healthy choices and give you useful tools and ideas, this book is not intended to replace parental wisdom and rules nor professional health and mental care. Be wise, as Molly knows you can be!

To Kat...for asking

PRAISE FOR MOLLY TOP

"This is the book I wish I had when I was a teen. Entertaining, honest, informative, and empowering, Molly Top demystifies love, sex, and everything in between."

—Daria Snadowsky, author of *Anatomy of a Boyfriend*

"If my mother had given me this book when I was an adolescent, I would have kept it to give to my daughter when she was a teen. Today's teens and moms desperately need the voice of Molly Top to advise and console. No bookstore should be without it, so it can be in every home!"

—Susan Krall, Owner
Off the Beaten Path
Bookstore, Coffeehouse and Bakery Café

CONTENTS

PROLOGUE

The microphone waits patiently to amplify my voice. I'm nervous because I'm about to give the valedictorian speech at my high school graduation and I'm pretty sure I'm going to offend some adults, maybe all of them.

"Hello!" I say enthusiastically.

"Hello!" the crowd cheers back. I like the feeling.

"It is our time!" I yell to my classmates. My fellow graduates scream and shout.

"We need to thank all of you family members and teachers and the administration for your love and support," I say like every other valedictorian is saying at every other high school graduation across the land, and I mean it. While I say the words I'm deciding if I have the guts to say the rest. I do, but I'd better warm them up some more.

"You've given us so much, and we're going to need it. We face some very difficult challenges, but you've given us most of the tools we'll need to do awesome things."

Everyone cheers again. I think they're ready.

"If you love your graduate, if you're proud of your graduate, STAND UP!" I demand.

The entire crowd gets to its feet clapping and cheering.

"Stay standing for a moment," I say. "You know," I act like I'm just coming up with this idea, "There is one thing I think we missed here in high school. There is one thing I think you could have done better."

The crowd waits for me to make my point, certain I will be amusing.

"I think you could have given us your wisdom in one area that would have helped us out a lot."

They grow restless waiting for what they are sure will be a joke or praise.

"So I have a little experiment."

Silence.

Then I say it. I say, "Sit down if you waited to have sex until marriage."

The stunned crowd remains standing.

"Yeah," I say, feeling bold. "Like 93% of you didn't wait."

I pause a full three seconds so this sinks in.

"Yet you taught us nothing else while we've been drowning in cyber sex and Internet porn. How crazy is that? We need so much more wisdom from you."

I look to my friends, my class, and say, "Let's change the course of our futures. Let's alter history. Let's have amazing sex lives."

A bunch of stuff happens at once. The microphone gets shut off. The standing crowd grumbles and sits in bewildered confusion. The principal comes up from behind and grabs my arm to escort me off the stage. My parents decide to return the new Prius they got me for graduation. The attending school board member decides to withhold my diploma. The journalist from the local paper wakes up and with a wicked smile begins writing like mad.

But the only important thing that happens is that my class-mates begin to wake up out of their sexual slumbers. My words ooze into their doped up minds. Slowly, a kid or two at a time stand and clap, then ten and twenty, then big chunks of my gown-clad peers rise, then every last kid stands and cheers, hands high above their heads. Many stand on their chairs.

They don't quite know why they are cheering. They just know there is a slight breeze of hope for our future. They don't know it is a future where soft, slow kisses satisfy way more that hook-ups, where we can discover great sex lives.

They just know something true is in the air.

Don't worry about me. Though I do drive a 1994 Corolla, I still got a full ride scholarship to my second-choice school. It was worth it.

PART 1

KNOW WHAT'S POSSIBLE

ONE

oh my god

Sex.

Sex, sex, sex, sex, sex, sex, sex!

Yeah, sex.

Let's declare a revolution on sex. Now. Big. Let's proclaim we will have great, amazing, fun, powerful, oh my god sex lives.

Let's do it differently than those before us.

Let's banish shame.

Let's banish guilt.

Let's banish insecurity.

Let's banish fear.

Let's really banish ignorance.

Let's learn from those who studied and mastered sex not only for pleasure, but for its ability to empower, to connect, to heal, to evoke awe, to open creativity, and to zoom us straight to the heavens.

Let's picture a future where we no longer act like eight-year-olds hiding our eyes when the prince kisses the girl. Let's not deny our own sexuality and in doing so open the gates of hell to porn, sexual abuses, and passionless marriages that lead to crazy divorce rates.

Yep, I blame all of this on immature views of sex.

Why am I writing this book? Because I can and I will. I'm Molly Top, age nineteen. I was valedictorian of my high school with a GPA of 4.33. I was the editor of my national award-winning high school newspaper, senior class president, and president of the National Honor Society. I got full-ride scholarship offers to Top Ten Schools.

I come from a good and loving family. We went to church every Sunday morning and Wednesday night. Until my senior year I'd only kissed one boy, badly.

My family clearly believes sex is for marriage and sexuality is to be put away until the wedding night. Oh, you can dress up for Homecoming and Prom. You can look sexy, but not slutty, and no sexy talk or lingering thoughts until "the night." After the vows and wedding cake, only then can you do it. Then you have a few kids and do it less and less.

I'd decided that teen sex was no fun, especially for girls. Too many of my friends told me about the sex they had and it sounded horrible. It sounded fast and unpleasant and unsatisfying. To make things worse, it seemed right after sex, the boys turned into emotional zombies and got as far away from the girls as possible. That was definitely not going to happen to me.

Anyway, last year I fell in love, love, love with Joe. We only had a few weeks together, but in that time my body and soul woke up. Woke up!!!

Joe was this confident, beautiful boy who loved me, loved himself, and loved our bodies and souls.

Holding hands with Joe was sexier, more erotic, and more arousing than most teen sex I'd heard about. Hell, it was sexier than any sex I'd heard about. We stared into each other's eyes. We kissed. God, did we kiss. We made out and our bodies tingled with an energy I didn't even know existed. We did a bunch of other stuff, too.

I wanted to do it all. ALL. My body didn't care about religion or marriage or anything. I wanted sex. Really wanted sex. Wanted Joe. All of him.

One night Joe smiled breathlessly between kisses after we'd walked all over town, making out at every secluded spot we could. This included picnic tables at the park, up against some trees, and on the dew-moistened grass by the lake. His hands were running up and down my back. I could feel his whole body pulse. I had just said, "I want to have sex with you."

"Oh, Molly," his mouth went against mine, tongue finding mine, hard.

Then he pulled back and stared into my eyes. His smile was amazing. His desire was amazing. I was so excited and terrified. I said to myself, *I'm gonna have sex. This is it. This is the moment.*

"It's not tonight," he said, as his hands pulled up my shirt so he could touch the skin of my back. His hands stopped just at the top of my jeans.

"It's not going to be me," he continued. "Not us."

I knew in an instant that he was right. I knew we weren't ready. I didn't really care because what was happening to my body under the zipper of my jeans was like nothing I'd ever thought could happen. All I wanted to do was have him touch me there. I didn't care with what.

I knew it wasn't going to happen that night, sex, but I was crazy with want, with desire for release. Joe rolled me over on my back and pressed his full weight on me. His pelvis was tense and hard, and as he kissed me he tilted himself into me. I tilted myself hard against him. Our mouths made this perfect circuit.

And then it happened.

I exploded. All that built-up want released in an explosion. I had my first orgasm. I moaned and arched my back and made

9

this guttural sound. I knew things right then. I knew I wasn't separate from anyone, anything. I knew my soul perfectly and realized it wasn't my resume. I knew Joe and I were one and we soared to heaven, to the cosmos somewhere. That huge pulsing took me to a place I've only experienced a few times in my life, but never like this. Never this rocket to total joy. This was perfect and huge.

Oh my God.

I didn't even try and contain my pleasure over this experience. I moaned and ground against Joe. Joe, who hadn't released, hadn't orgasmed.

Then it began to fade. I quickly left heaven and returned to my body under Joe's.

I was amazed and exposed and not excited or aroused any longer. I felt incredibly close to Joe. I loved him so much.

He smiled at me. He was so happy, so dear. He rolled off me, which I appreciated because I was so relaxed. So done.

I knew he wasn't, but he wasn't angry or demanding more. I could see he was breathing deeply, pulling away from his passion and his desire for release.

I loved this man. Loved him.

"I can't believe what happened," I said to Joe.

He smiled. "Amazing."

"Joe, this is something."

"Yes."

"I love you."

"We love each other."

I could have felt stupid and exposed, but I was with Joe. I felt loved and peaceful. But more than all that, I felt like I'd discovered something no one had ever told me about. Like I had a million dollars in a bank account I could access any time. I realized sex isn't some dirty thing, some sin, something we do only to have kids.

Sex isn't the hump. It isn't the frantic, empty stuff you see on TV. It isn't what happens at parties where everyone is drunk. It isn't something we do to prove our worth or prove we're not gay. It isn't social status.

No.

I realized sex is a huge gift from whatever creative force built this life of ours. Sex is a huge part of our spiritual world, our desire for connection, our search for meaning and purpose. Besides all that, it is so normal and natural, like breathing and smiling.

I'd just figured out that sex is a glorious gift, and I, Molly Top, was going to find out everything about it. I was going to discover why no one had told me about it. I was going to uncover why most teen sex was so bad, so not what I just experienced.

I'm smart. I write well. I research like a mad woman.

I interviewed teens and adults about their sex lives—not just about intercourse (crappy word!), but about their entire romantic and sexual lives. I asked about great sex and bad sex. I asked about relationships. I asked about orgasms (great word!). I got my brother, Jo Sha (a.k.a., Joshua), to interview guys because it got too awkward when I tried.

I looked up articles on healthy, happy sexuality and found entirely different ways of looking at sex. I found ancient teachings that saw sexuality as a sacred art form. These transformed my entire view on sex. They gave me hope for our future.

I'm not a slut. I'm not a whore. I have simply become an expert on teen sexuality and on the ancient teachings on the art of sex.

I am committed to our generation creating a better life than the one being handed us.

Why sex?

Because I believe it is a driving force for change. I also believe it has been a driving force for oppression, making us feel bad about ourselves, making us fear our bodies and desires. I believe older, more advanced cultures studied and mastered sexuality. They left us directions, like treasure maps. I think the landscape has changed, but we can find it and then use it in our way, in our time.

I believe what I said in my valedictorian speech: We do face difficult challenges. We need to be as healthy and creative and self-confident as possible. We need great sex lives.

TWO

clicking the switch

Remember when kissing on TV made you sick? When any member of the opposite sex made you sick? When you first learned about doing *it* made you sick? When everything you learned about doing *it* made you sick?

Remember?

Remember when some older kid, or later some friend suddenly got interested in *it*? Talked about *it* more? Did something like hold hands or kiss or make out? Remember how kids loved to tell stories about all sorts of kids doing all sorts of things including *it*?

Remember how *it* scared you, grossed you out, and angered you because of how wrong *it* was?

Maybe you're still there, but if you're reading this, your switch has probably already clicked, or at least it's twitching.

You then went from horrified to curious. From a body that went cold at such thoughts to a body that grew warm with such thoughts, that squirmed with such thoughts. A body that could stop concentrating on school or family or friends or anything in order to ponder all the aspects of *it*, of romance, of sexuality, of sex itself.

This happens at different times for different kids. Some kids are young when their switch clicks, some are pretty old. Some switches click huge, some start slow and build huge, some click and stay rather mild.

Regardless, the switch does click, and in one of a zillion ways you go from sexually asleep to wide awake. You go from thinking there's no way you'll ever do anything as disgusting as *it* to someone who is pretty sure you will.

Know this, every adult's switch clicked on at one time or another. Just like yours did. Adults and kids often forget this.

Now, the clicking of the sexual switch should be an amazing time, but it's often a time of great conflict and pain. It didn't used to be that way. Not so far back in history when we hit this age of our switch clicking, we married. We married young in perfect timing with our bodies.

We married at the ages of fifteen to nineteen, right when our bodies are dying to have sex. But we became more "civilized" and we postponed the appropriate age of marriage so that we'd be older and better parents, better educated, better financially prepared to start families. And we postponed and we postponed. Now the average age of marriage in our culture is twenty-seven for men and twenty-five for women.

So, here we have these bodies designed by God himself with switches clicked full on, and we're supposed to wait and wait for five, ten, fifteen years?

Tension mounts.

Rules are made. Adults, who have obviously forgotten all this, make more and more rules. They tell us to put our sexuality out of our minds. (Like they did!) They tell us to abstain (like they did!), but they give us no alternatives. Nothing.

Our sex education consists only of the medical mechanics of sex, the possible horrid consequences of sex, like STDs and unwanted pregnancies, and lectures on abstinence-only. It's taught

14

right alongside drug education, like it's something bad. No wonder we're all messed up about it.

Look at the pathetic state of teen sex in our culture. We have both huge abstinence-only messages and huge pornography influence. Sex is everywhere: every ad, our clothes, movies (even PG-13), TV (naked butts and full-on sex), and mother-of-all-porn dispensers, the Internet.

So adults are screaming "Don't do it, but swim in it while you wait."

Well guess what? Our sex, our generation's sex, sucks (and not just literally!). Sex in our culture is some of the least evolved, interesting, mature, loving, or spiritual of any culture. I know this because I asked.

According to the teens I interviewed, our sex is fast, uncreative, and unsatisfying. Yet many teens are certainly having sex. Eighty percent of us will have sex before we're twenty. 80%! That's a lot more than most of us! So we're having sex. We're having bad sex, and no one is giving us honest advice. No one is giving us true wisdom, wisdom that admits sex is a strong and potentially great force in every human's life.

Where are the answers to the real questions we have, like what is good sex like? How do girls have orgasms? How do you know your body is ready for sex? How do you know if you're ready for sex? How do you feel connected sexually? How do you go from kissing to intercourse (what a horrid word!)? How do you not feel stupid afterwards? How do you honor your body and its desires and honor your parents and your community and God?

THREE

mindful sex

Mindful sex is sexuality that isn't just something a body does without thought, like burping or nose picking, but something one masters like playing an instrument or making an amazing meal. Older civilizations had schools of thought that taught people how to transform mindless sexuality into an art form. They called them the sacred sexual arts. Tantric sex and *The Kama Sutra* are the best known, most published, and easiest to access.

They all say basically the same thing: sex is a sacred art.

Think about that. First, sex is sacred. Why? Is it? Most of the stories I hear about actual intercourse don't seem too sacred.

What does sacred mean anyway? My dictionary says it means "declared holy." Declared holy? Right up there with church, communion, Christmas, and baptism? Aren't they all declared holy?

How can fumbling around in the back seat of your car be holy? How can a drunken make-out session at a party be holy?

Holy, "associated with divine power."

Divine power.

I know most people hear sex and power and think whips and chains, but really, sexuality itself, mastered, produces power. At least that's what other cultures believe. In fact, in the ancient civilizations of India, Japan, and China the sexual arts were

16

considered secrets known only by royalty, the wealthy, and the powerful. They didn't want the servants, the common people, knowing them. They needed a class of powerless people.

Powerless people. How sexy are they?

So can you become powerful through sexuality? Oh, yeah, because I swear to you *The Matrix* was right. We're all copper-tops, batteries, producers of electricity, of energy, of power. We can be weak, cheap batteries, or never-ending, always-fully-charged batteries.

To be fully charged we need great circuitry that flows without obstacles. This circuitry needs to be flowing well inside us so it can flow to and from others. Things like nature, beauty, inspired thoughts, laughter, creativity, joy, and love help a lot. Flow and recharging can certainly come from mastered sexuality.

Yet that isn't the kind of sexuality teens are experiencing. I hear kids talk about sex like it was something they own, they collect. Kind of like "I *got* to go to Hawaii," "I *got* so high," and "I *got* these really cute jeans," or "I *got* laid."

Got.

Huh. There's no flow in *got.*

But if someone talks about what came before *got*, what they say does seem holy, not *got.*

Attraction. Eyes meet. Shy smiles exchanged. Talk about nothing while bodies talk, decide. Move closer. Touch, lean into, shove a little, tickle, wrestle. See the best in the other, that person of desire. Connect. Eyes, then maybe hands. Arm around shoulder, around a waist. Lean into. Eyes. Smiles. Lick of the lips. Body wide awake. Smile. Eyes.

That beginning, the things you say, the way you think, the kindness, the tenderness, the fun, the play, the connections, and most important, the way you see the dazzling soul in the other and in yourself, *that* my friends is holy.

From here we don't seem to know where to go. So we go from holy to *got* and lose the wonder. It is in the space between holy and *got* that so much pain occurs in relationships.

But, it doesn't have to be that way.

The sacred sexual arts teach ways of mastering one's sexuality to eliminate the pain that occurs between holy and *got*.

That's the art form.

Tantric texts speak of the Sixty-Four Sacred Arts. These are everyday art forms, many of which don't cost much and don't need years of formal instruction. Tantric teaching believes if you bring some of these into your life, your life will be enriched with beauty, peace, harmony, joy, healing, connectedness, generosity, and great balance. You'll be fully charged and your energy will flow well.

According to the texts, sex is the one art form we all must study. We may choose from the rest. The Sixty-Four Sacred Arts include singing, dancing, music, writing, drawing, painting, sewing, reading, poetry, physical sports, sculpture, gymnastics, games, flower arranging, cooking, decoration, gardening, languages, etiquette, carpentry, magic, chemistry, mineralogy, architecture, religious rites, household management, disguise, and martial arts, and more.

What a different way of thinking about sex. Revolutionary, really. To think of sex as something to be studied, practiced, and mastered. This would involve patience, focus, and alertness. Otherwise it's just squeaking out notes on a violin like first-year players do in middle school. It's fun enough but not beautiful. It enriches your life very little and enriches others less.

And you certainly don't start off playing duets!

FOUR

connection

If sex is an art form, then connection is the medium. Connection becomes the acrylics to paint with, the notes to play, the ink to create the words.

It's all about connection.

My favorite greeting goes like this: put your palms together and bow slightly. The other person does the same. Then you say "Namaste" (pronounced nah-mah-stay) to one another. It means, loosely translated, "The divine in me acknowledges the divine in you."

Can you imagine what our sex lives would be like if before each embrace, each kiss, each sexual act along the way to sex, we acknowledged the divine in the other.

Talk about connection.

It may sound corny and unrealistic, but isn't that what the first moments of attraction are all about? Aren't we seeing the best, the divine, in the other? Aren't we really saying, "The best in me acknowledges the best in you?" or "The soul in me sees the soul in you?" Or "The sexy beast in me acknowledges the sexy beast in you?"

Sometimes when I'm racing through the halls at school, I make myself stop and watch everyone. I look at the blank faces trying to pretend they don't need connection, yet I think we are thirsty for connection, for divine connection. If I happen to catch someone's eyes, I smile a smile that tells them I see the divine in them. It's magic. They light up.

I think we're standing in a river of connection, yet we're dying of thirst. Here are all these glorious souls we can connect with, but we just pass them by, not knowing we could drink. Not knowing we never have to be thirsty again. Never alone.

Our habit is to disconnect. We are quick to gossip, hate, fear, and create drama and chaos. We get distracted by our huge want of everything. We would rather be entertained than connected (I blame this entirely on *Barney*).

All we have to do is stop and see the divine in ourselves and the other.

Then we can paint!

Mary Pipher, author of *Reviving Ophelia*, writes in her book *Writing to Change the World*, "If I have one great idea, it is that connecting people might save the world." How we connect with others sexually is a huge part of how we connect in general. Isn't sex the ultimate connection?

What the hell is connection anyway?

This gets back to the fact that we are all energy, and energy can only move, can only be powerful, through connection. That's why we have to plug computers into walls. That's why wires hang across our towns and under the grounds of our cities.

Electricity moves from source to source.

Have you ever seen those electric balls sold in science stores or those specialty shops that sell T-shirts you can't wear at school? They're like globes of electrical current. If you touch them, the current finds your hand. It seeks you out. It doesn't hurt, but you can feel it. I own one of these and touch it all the time, just to remind me of what's happening between all of us all the time, only we can't see it.

If you can, imagine that every minute we're sending out those tentacles of electricity, like little lightning bolts. Then, when we're near others, we connect electrically. The closer we get, the greater the potential for connection.

Not all connection is warm and fuzzy and sexy. We all know this; that's why we choose not to connect.

The main forms of connection are: (1) weak and dull connections (boring), (2) the ones where we try and take the energy from the other (yuck!), and (3) the kind where together our joined energy creates bigger and greater energy (amazing!). We plug into the huge energy that created the oceans, the cosmos, us!

FIVE

the big O

Which brings us to the Big O, the Big Bang. Yep, the orgasm.

Enlightened adults may say, "Orgasm is not the primary goal of sex," but, come on, it is the goal of sex.

Release as it is called in the sacred arts.

Release after a great build-up.

I love the term orgasm. It's the only sexual term that is beautiful and perfectly descriptive. It sounds just like what occurs during an orgasm. You build and build and build with tension and excitement. You expand and expand. You go beyond the confines of your body. Your internal circuitry begins firing at an enormous rate. And though the energy starts to focus in your groin, it radiates out through your torso, your fingertips, down your thighs straight to your feet.

In tantric sex, one uses the orgasm as a way to begin mastering one's sexuality.

First and foremost, you don't learn about orgasm from someone else. You learn it from yourself.

Most kids I interviewed reported that once their switch clicked, they thought they should immediately go have sex. Many did. Most said the experience was a letdown. This seemed true especially for the girls. There was almost no foreplay, because the goal was to have sex, to de-virginize, to find out what it was about.

Having sex soon after your switch has clicked is like trying to play a solo at Carnegie Hall right after you get your first violin. It's gonna be bad, really bad.

We don't learn to have sex by having sex. Kids and adults who had bad early sexual experiences said although they've had some okay sex later, they still don't see that sex is all that great. They seem to be eternally disappointed by it.

We learn about great sex by exploring our sexuality ourselves. We learn sex by studying sex. We learn sex by knowing ourselves. Do not let anyone but yourself teach you about your body. You could end up feeling resentful, disappointed, embarrassed, and alone. These are not the feelings sex is supposed to bring.

I know this sounds hypocritical because I certainly never had an orgasm before my night with Joe, but that was unusual. I'm also fairly certain if we'd had sex that night, it wouldn't have been good. Up until then, I didn't know my body or sexuality at all. Now I do. Now I'm an expert.

So first, know thyself.

Yes, I'm talking about masturbation. (I apologize for the word masturbation. I won't use it again. It sounds medical. It conjures the sound of purple plastic gloves being snapped into place before some horrid procedure. I'll use the term *self-pleasure* from now on.)

It's pretty clear that almost every boy can self-pleasure. It's also pretty clear they have no clue there are many ways to self-pleasure. I believe this is the beginning of bad future sex. The goal so clearly becomes the orgasm that speed and disconnection become the habit of how to get there. We'll go into this later, but for now, boys, consider self-pleasure as the groundwork for great future sex.

Self-pleasure for girls is more complicated. In my interviews I found that girls don't want to talk about this topic. It seems some girls do self-pleasure, but plenty don't. Some didn't know what I was talking about. Some had tried with no luck, no orgasm. Many thought the idea too embarrassing and gross to even try. Interesting, too embarrassing or gross? I mean having sex with some random guy you met an hour ago can really be embarrassing and gross.

Doctors will tell you (but you probably won't ask) that there are health benefits to self-pleasure, such as providing a healthy outlet for people who choose to abstain, allowing people to get to know their sexual bodies, reducing stress, helping you sleep, and encouraging self esteem. So there!

Religions and belief systems differ widely on sex, sexuality, and self-pleasure, yet few even discuss orgasm. It's in the where and with whom and when that gets regulated. None specifically deny that the orgasm is one great gift from God, Allah, the Goddess, whatever.

Know your beliefs and make decisions from there about self-pleasure. Should you decide practicing self-pleasure is a way to master sexuality, there is an exercise in Chapter 13. (Can you believe it?)

PART 2

KNOW THE BASES

SIX

the batter's box

There are hundreds of amazing steps from attraction to sex.
Each step requires a decision.

"This is fantastic. I want to stay here."

"This is too far. I want to go back a step."

"This is too far. I want to stop."

"This is amazing. I want to go to the next step."

Or, in our sex world, "This is nice. I want to skip sixty steps
and have sex." Ugh!

I'm spending a third of this book on the steps that can and
should precede actual sex.

If you believe what teens say or what the sacred sexual texts
say, then the main reason our sex lives are marginal is because
we don't take our time. We skip most of the steps. We don't allow ourselves the time to connect emotionally and energetically.
We don't even know there are steps. Hell, we don't even know we
have the possibility for great sex lives.

All sacred sex teachings emphasize that the body is perfectly
created for sexuality. There is a process, a natural progression
that leads to great sex. Our bodies unfold to sex.

For this section on the steps towards sex, I decided to use the
old standard baseball metaphor: First Base, Second Base, Third
Base, and of course, the Home Run.

Ancient tantric teachers would roll over in their graves if they
thought I was taking all the steps down to four. I'm not. I am

simply categorizing these steps into four: attraction, touching, intimate touching, and sex.

Besides, I love baseball.

I love the smell of the dirt, the sound of the bat cracking after a perfectly hit ball, the taste of roasted peanuts. I like the slow pace of the game because it's all about how you get from here to there. I like the fit of those uniforms, too.

For some reason, baseball bases have been the metaphor for stages of sexuality for decades. Sex isn't a game. Not really. It certainly isn't a matter of stealing bases. I'm still going to use the metaphor because ball players inspire me.

I added The Batter's Box because tantric teaching emphasizes that before you begin your romantic and sexual life with others you must prepare yourself. Certainly learning to self-pleasure and to self-pleasure well is part of that preparation. Even more important, you just have to like yourself if you're going to have a good sex life. I guess you've got to like yourself if you're going to have a good life of any kind.

The Batter's Box. Love yourself. How? There's so much we think that makes us not like ourselves. We don't like how we look. We don't like how we act, what we say, or how we do anything from school work to taking out the trash.

We've spent our lives hearing what we aren't, and now we believe it. Mostly what we hear from parents, teachers, peers, TV, movies, advertisers is that we simply aren't good enough. We hear it so much we eventually feel like we aren't good enough to exist. We feel purposeless and powerless. How sexy is that?

One of the few things in life that sparks us up, makes us think maybe we're of some value, is attraction. There is nothing like being attracted to someone who is attracted back.

Nothing.

This can be the attraction of friends, adults who see potential in us, and then, of course, a possible romantic or sexual interest. Let's face it, at our age, that's the attraction that we adore.

The more we like ourselves, the more others are attracted to us. Simple as that.

So, how do you feel about yourself? Are you worthy of breathing the air? Do you add to anyone's life? Are you beautiful? Do you create beauty? Does your existence enhance this world?

In case you're wondering, the answer to all these questions is "Hell yes!!!"

Try it, "Hell yes!!!"

Take a piece of paper and fold it in half. On one half write all the negative things you say about yourself. You know them, "I'm fat, lazy, stupid, ugly, boring, annoying, a loser..." Know them, don't deny them. Those thoughts are banging around your head every day anyway. Then, on the other side write down the opposites, "I'm perfect, motivated, smart, beautiful, interesting, fun..." Got it?

Stop saying the negative and replace them with the positive. Stop believing the negative and start believing the positive. These negative thoughts take a long time to shift to the positive, but if you stick to it they do indeed shift.

There may be some realistic things you want to change. When it comes to sexuality we usually focus on our bodies. Like middle-aged adults who have become overweight and flabby, kids report they sometimes avoid their sexuality because of their bodies. But we aren't middle-aged. We're young and should be all about being sexy.

The tantric teaching go over specific ways of living that enhance our self-confidence and therefore enhance our sexuality.

Simple things.

Hygiene. Brush your teeth, your tongue, and floss (I added that one. They didn't have floss back then). Wash well, every crevasse. Wear clean clothes. Smell good, and not like you're wearing a gallon of some cologne like SAW or Au d'Popstar.

Get outside. Walk. Go into nature. Nature is sexy. Get some sun, some exercise. We feel sexier when we've been near beauty, near wonder.

Laugh, especially with others, not at them. Laughing is sexy. Really. Laughing is a way to remember how connected we are, which reminds us of our worth. Laugh.

Connect with those whose confidence is strong, not weak. People with weak self-confidence pull you down. Teenagers in general have weak self-confidence. They pull each other down. Find strong friends. Find strong adults. Find plants, animals, and young children. They never doubt themselves. That's why it's great being around them. Connecting is sexy.

Be creative. Practice some of the Sixty-Four Sacred Arts. You'll see your own wonder in beauty, in inspiration, in creativity. Creativity is sexy.

Eat well. Fast foods, salty foods, fatty foods, sugary foods are not sexy. They make you fat and lazy. Cook and eat meals. Eat more veggies, grains, and fruit. Have dinners with your family and your friends. Healthy skin, hair, and bodies are sexy.

Stop watching TV and playing video games all the time. (I added this one, too.) They turn you into middle-aged slugs. Staring at a screen, pushing buttons is not sexy. Wasting years of your life in front of a screen steals your sexuality. Remember, the wealthy need a dull and obedient working class, a people without power. Don't become those people. They aren't sexy.

Be healthy, active, creative, and you will know your worth and you'll be attractive. Now it's time to step up to the plate and swing away.

SEVEN

first base

So now that you're all confident (don't even think about going to first base unless you know your worth), you're ready to notice and act upon your attractions.

First Base. Attraction. We're attracted to a lot of people a lot of the time. We're attracted all the time to someone—somebody on TV, in a movie, some kid in math class (hell, some kid in any class), our neighbor, our good "friend," pretty much anybody.

So how does this broad attraction focus onto just one person? Who knows, but it does. For some it happens daily, for some it happens just a handful of times in their lives. One moment you're attracted to someone, the next you are attracted to a person who is attracted to you and both of you know it. Now the fun begins.

Somehow you and that person are face to face, or ear to phone, or eye to screen—regardless, you and the other are going to exchange words. Maybe you're already friends. Maybe you've never met.

Anyway, attraction leads to engagement (no, not like a wedding). One of you speaks to the other. The words are lame, like, "Hey, wassup?" "Not much." "I see you in biology class." "You're on the volleyball team, right?" Blah, blah, blah.

What's really being said is between the bodies. "Hey, I think you're hot." "I've been thinking about you for a long time." "You think I'm hot?" "You noticed me before?" "You won't hurt me, right?" "God, I want to touch your hair, kiss your neck."

Right then, at that silent thought, the other, the object of attraction, throws back her beautiful hair and exposes her neck, even though in real talk she just said, "You're on the volleyball team, right?"

Weird, huh? With attraction and engagement, words go out the window and unspoken communication becomes loud. Sometimes everyone in the room can hear.

So, depending on the circumstances, you'll either keep this going or move apart. For example, if you're at someone's house and curfew is hours away, you'll keep it going. If you just had a few minutes in study hall and the bell rings, the moment has passed, but the door is now open. Using my baseball metaphor, you hit a single.

You made it to first base. The door is open. You both are attracted and you're engaging each other. No touch, maybe a playful shove or wrestle, but there's been no commitment of romance or sexuality. No kiss, no handhold.

As with ball players, most sexual encounters don't get past first base. Still, first base is a blast. Hopefully you make it to first base a zillion times in your life.

Unspoken communication, possibility, searching for the best in another, eyes meeting, flirting, feeling great about yourself, hope, promise...ah yes, first base, the base of possibility.

In the movie *Crouching Tiger, Hidden Dragon* this couple has loved each other all their lives yet they never move off first base. They respect the man's role as a warrior who is not allowed to be in a romantic relationship. There is one scene where he simply reaches over and touches her hand. It is one of the most romantic moments in a movie, and it all takes place on first base.

At the moment of a purposeful touch, a kiss, a handhold, an arm around the waist, a hug with a kiss to the top of the head or neck, then—and only then—do you advance to second base.

EIGHT

second base

This is the base most often skipped by our generation. One girl put it so perfectly, "You make out first. You don't kiss until after you make out. You kiss only if you really like someone."

"But you can make out with just anyone?"

"Oh yeah, kissing is more intimate."

How screwed up is that?

I like kissing.

I like kissing a lot.

There is a scene in the movie *What Women Want* when a date consists just of an amazingly long kissing scene. Another good kissing scene is in *The Lake House* after a great dance scene. Really, they'll make you swoon. Make a list of your favorite kissing scenes from movies to remind you why great kisses are vital to great relationships. Never ever compromise on a kiss.

Best second base story. This woman about fifty told me this one.

I was on the Amtrak from Chicago to Washington D.C.. I'd just graduated from college. I was in the lounge car and this very attractive guy was playing cards with an older couple.

So I joined the card game. We played for hours late into the night. We were obviously very attracted to each other. We laughed a lot, both of us being clever and funny. The older couple was enjoying the heck out us. Then I felt his foot on mine. I grabbed his foot between my feet. He grabbed back. I took off my shoes. So did he. So there we were playing hardcore footsie under the table while playing cards above the table. I can't tell you how erotic feet can be. I hadn't had sex before. And even though I'd done a lot of sexual stuff with guys, I'd never had anything this sexually exciting.

We rubbed feet together like lovers for hours. When we finally ended the game he followed me to my seat and sat next to me. We kissed until the sun came up and Washington D.C. drew near.

I never saw him again, but that was the most fun I ever had staying on second base in my life.

Second base. Holding hands, embracing, kissing, French kissing, hands up and down the back, breasts pressed against chests, pelvis rubbing against pelvis, clothing always between flesh. Lots of non-verbal stuff going on.

Bodies wake up. Groins get hard or wet, pulse, want to press against the other.

Lots of dancing is second base sort of sexuality. Holding waists, grinding against the other, kissing necks, kissing mouths, pelvis finding pelvis like magnets.

Second base is the base we teens need to know about, honor, master, and linger on.

Second base. You have a slightly better chance at getting home from second base than from first. But more than likely you'll spend the whole inning there. You should have a blast while you wait.

The art form to second base is in the lingering. It is in the body slowly building in excitement, then slowing down. It is in the nibbled ear, the kiss on the top of the head, the forehead touching the forehead. The divine acknowledging the divine.

You could say, "I'm staying at second base for a long time... 'til I'm eighteen, 'til I'm married, 'til I'm in love."

Remember, the excitement that begins building on second base can be released without having sex. You can go to the privacy of your own bed, then recall the experience on second base, and self-pleasure to great satisfaction. You can also practice the art of calming down the energy created on second base and using it for something else like doing any of the other Sixty-Four Sacred Arts.

Remember this.

You need to linger at second base a long time to know how you feel about the person you are with. Besides being attracted, ask yourself do you like this person? Do you respect this person? Does he/she try and go too fast, too slow? Does he/she have any mastery over their sexuality? Spend time with that person. Are they kind? What sorts of relationships have they had in the past? Can you talk about sexuality with them? Are they self-confident? Do they like you or do they simply want to get you? Be honest about how attracted you are as you play on second base. How's the kissing? What's happening to your body?

I'd never go further than second base unless I'd gone there many times with someone. I mean it. Go to second base again and again with someone until you know if you want to go further. The next bases are significantly more vulnerable. Your trust needs to be very high. Your feelings about going further need to be very strong.

This woman in college I interviewed told me this story about making a decision about a boy by his response to their time on second base.

My very first boyfriend, my very first kiss was this boy, this very popular, hot, six-packed athlete-of-the-week kind of guy. I was not very popular or hot or a great athlete. We knew each other from our church youth group. This church had clearly taught we shouldn't do anything but hold hands until we got married. Lots of our friends got married at seventeen and eighteen years of age just so they could have sex.

Well, I'd gone out with this boy for a few months. I liked him a lot. We'd kissed. We'd made out a few times. Then one night, at a drive-in, we were making out and he pulled me over to him so that I was straddling him, sitting on his lap, facing him.

We were definitely pelvis to pelvis, kissing. I had no idea how fun this making out could be. I trusted him and myself, completely. We kissed. We rubbed against each other and then his hands found my breasts, over my shirt, over my bra.

It was so fun, so nice.

And then, the next day, he asked if he could meet with me. He told me he thought we'd sinned. He said he thought we should pray for forgiveness.

At first I was embarrassed. I mean, this kid was better looking than me, more sought after sexually. He was a star jock for god's sake. Having him for a boyfriend certainly had improved my social status.

But then he said we'd sinned.

I realized I completely disagreed with him. I didn't think we'd sinned. I thought we'd had a blast. I thought we had been very respectful of each other. I thought we knew each other well, knew our bodies well.

So I told him this and I broke up with him. I wasn't going to judge myself harshly for being loving and adventurous and careful and true to myself.

Looking back, he might have been scared we were heading towards early sex. He might have been right.

I know I didn't get another serious boyfriend for another five years. I dated, kissed, but stayed away from heavy petting.

A man told me about his first date with the woman who is now his wife.

We went to an animation festival. In the dark of the theater I took her hand and held it for about an hour. Then I began rubbing it with my thumb. I wanted her to know how much I liked her. We touched fingertips, interlocked fingers. Finally, I brought her hand to my lips. I turned it so I could kiss her palm, right in the middle. She pulled our hands to her mouth. Then she put one of the tips of my fingers into her mouth. I'll always remember that moment. I went crazy. It felt amazing. That's all we did that night. Hold and kiss hands. That's how I knew I'd marry her. We still spend a lot of time holding and kissing hands.

Our sex lives will be revolutionized if we learn to linger at second. This is the base of knowing the other. Don't skip it. Don't simply tag the base and sprint to third. Build the excitement. Let your body get aroused. Back away from the arousal. Let it get aroused again and again.

At some point you will feel safe and comfortable. You will have decided you're ready to go further. You'll grab your partners hand and you'll head to third base.

NINE

third base

Ah...third base.

In a mindful world, we'd linger at first and go to second only if we're completely comfortable with ourselves and the other. We'd enjoy second to its fullest. We'd allow our bodies to enjoy without forcing, without rushing. We'd use second base to deepen our connection, and build our desire and excitement, while being honest about the other, the circumstances, the timing and safety.

If all is well, we'd jog over to third.

Third base, unlike its baseball metaphor, requires fewer clothes than the first two bases. Inhibitions disappear. Hands, tongues, mouths explore the other to a tremendous building of excitement and want.

Many guys and girls reported they'd like to play at third. They'd like to try stuff without assuming they'd go all the way. They'd like to go forward and backward. They'd like to take care of their own release or release without actual sex.

You know, they'd like to orgasm without actual sex. They'd like to orgasm by grinding into each other, by hands, fingers, by oral sex. They'd like to do everything but have intercourse, but this doesn't seem as acceptable as it did in the past. Almost every kid I interviewed thought if you went to third base you were obligated to go Home. You aren't.

Until recently teens fooled around a lot, but most didn't have actual sex. They did "everything but..." I interviewed a lot of adults who said they tried so many things for months and even years. Overall, they reported they had far better sex lives than teens report these days. They reported their first actual sex was far, far better than the first actual sex of teens today. Why? Because they went slowly through the bases and got to know their bodies. They knew exactly when they were ready to have sex, and they still waited a long time.

I've heard adults complain that so many kids are having oral sex in order to avoid having actual intercourse. I'm not sure why so many adults have a problem with oral sex. Stats would say most sexually active adults have tried, if not continue to have, oral sex. I say if both or either partner like having it and giving it, then that is the couple's choice.

I interviewed many girls who had given oral sex. Some of them liked it. They thought it was fun and enjoyed it a lot. They felt safer about oral sex than actual sex because they didn't want to get pregnant. Some had felt pressured and hated it. A lot of girls enjoyed the action but did not want the boy to orgasm in their mouths. So say that. Tell your partner what you are willing to do and what you aren't. Set it up ahead of time.

I know there is a chance of getting sexually transmitted diseases through oral sex. Again, that's why you don't go anywhere near third unless you know your partner really well. You know if and who they've been with. You should know their safety and yours. (See Chapter 14.)

Mindful sex is a pattern of first base to a slow second to a very slow third, back to first. Build then recede, back and forth. So if you're going to mess around, if you're gonna play ball, if you want to master sex, then practice. Have a partner you can practice with. Talk directly about going forward. Easing off. Talk about how far is the furthest you want to go. Master your desire. Master your excitement.

Important note: just because your partner wants to go to second or third or home doesn't mean you want to. I heard both girls and boys say they were shocked when their partner took off a piece of their clothing or the other's clothing.

Practice how to say "I'm not comfortable with that." "I don't know you that well." "I want to know you better." Or simply, "No."

It isn't easy saying *No* in the middle of a serious make-out session. It isn't easy hearing the other ways partners say *No* with their bodies. Third base is for when you are old enough and mature enough to know if you want to say *No*, to say *No* when you need to, and to know when your partner is silently saying *No*.

There are signs that your partner is saying *No* without using words. These are a little embarrassing to talk about, but they are really important. One of the first signs your partner is saying *No* is that they are not moving forward with you. You are moving them forward. They are not pulling your body to theirs, they stop initiating kissing, they are not removing their clothes, they are not smiling or laughing or talking or making "mmmmm" noises. They have grown silent and cold. They are not initiating anything any longer. They are like rag dolls.

(Get ready, because like third base, this part is Rated R.)

The most obvious and least talked about non-verbal *No, I'm not ready* sign for boys is that their penises are not hard and for girls that their vaginas are not lubricated. These are absolute clear signs that your partner is not ready to be doing whatever you are doing. Stop. Put your clothes back on. Figure out why you weren't ready, like maybe you're too young (remember you have to be 18 to see a rated-R movie), maybe you don't really like or trust the person you are with, maybe you are feeling guilty, maybe you haven't been playing ball long enough.

Note: Just because a penis is hard and a vagina is wet does not mean the partner is saying *Yes*, but if it isn't hard or wet then it is a definite *NO!!!!*

I heard terrible stories from girls where in the first few minutes into kissing, the boy put his hands down the girl's pants and stuck his fingers into her very dry vagina. Here she's barely on second base and he's acting like they're on third and it hurt and was no fun at all. The girls felt violated. Some stopped the whole thing. Some kept going because they thought if the boy had his finger in her she was obligated to go all the way. She wasn't!!!

A lot of girls believe that sexy girls are ready for anything, anytime. They believe sexy girls don't say *No*. They are so wrong. Really sexy girls love their bodies and their sexuality and they will say *No* anytime things are just not right.

If you are with a partner worthy of any romantic and sexual encounter they will join you in some talk.

"Is this okay?"

"What would you like to do?"

"Can I try this?"

Not just the basic, "Oh baby, you're so sexy."

Or "I love you." (And you just met.)

Or "I want you so bad."

Third base is tricky. Be safe. Be careful. Be sure of yourself. Be sure of your ability to stop when and where you want to stop. Be sure you trust your partner.

Be sure because a Home Run is just 90 feet away.

TEN

home run

It's pretty simple. Traditionally: penis in vagina. (Gay mechanics are a bit modified, but it's the same idea).

Look at pictures from tantric texts or from *The Kama Sutra*. You can see them online or at any bookstore. The ancient drawings are explicit with the penis in the vagina, yet the faces are calm, the eyes focused on the other. The pace is not frantic. It is beautiful.

Until sex can be like that, don't do it. Practice. Have fun. Self-pleasure, but don't have bad sex. Bad sex can taint your whole future sex life.

If you ever look at porn you'll see neither partner ever looks at the other. There is no tenderness, no respect, and no joy. The goal is quick self-pleasure, usually at the expense of the other.

If you can't stare into the eyes of your partner, clean and clear, full of desire, respect, love, joy, creativity, honesty, guilt-free, then don't do it. Because someday you will be able to.

A movie that depicts fast, unloving sex, skipping second and third base, is *8 Mile*. The couple has had a moment of attraction. They find themselves with an opportunity to have sex. So they find a private place. He lifts up her skirt while he kisses her. She licks her palm to lubricate herself. They then have a thirty-second sexual encounter. They never look at each other. A day later he finds her having sex with his business partner.

A great sex scene is in this old movie called *Say Anything*. Even though the sex occurs in the back seat of a car, the couple is certain of their actions. They are respectful, responsible. They stare deeply into each other's eyes.

Here's a home run checklist:

How long have you known each other?

How sober are you?

Are you able to talk about what might happen?

How safe is the environment?

How safe is your body?

Can you look into the eyes of the other?

How aroused is your body? Is it ready?

What does your inner voice say?

How will you feel after?

If you've scored a home run, I hope it was good. I hope you really loved your partner. I hope you had an amazing orgasm. I hope you were so responsible you know your body is safe. I hope you're still smiling big. I hope this is the beginning of a fabulous sex life. A fabulous life.

If not, no worries. Stop. Go back to the beginning, back to the Batter's Box, and slowly become a master. It's not over. Heal up. Take your time. Use the experience to do it differently. Slowly. Do not, really, *do not* keep having sex just because you've had sex once. Don't stay with the partner if it was bad. If you don't really like that person anymore, don't force the relationship. It seldom gets better. Sex is too intimate to compromise.

The sensitivity and delicacy of the skin in the vagina melded with the sensitivity of the penis makes sex so vulnerable. Condom in-between or not. It's not like any of the other bases. It's not like holding hands. Bodies are interlocked. Fluids are enter-

44

ing each other on a cellular level. New electrical currents are made. Sex is amazing. Honor it. Master it. As the wise character, Cher, says in *Clueless*, "You know how picky I am about my shoes, and they only go on my feet."

Part 3

Know the Rest

ELEVEN

flirting

I am starting out this *Know the Rest* section with a chapter on flirting because I believe flirting is one of the best things in life. Flirting is one of the most fun parts of life. You can't talk about The Rest without talking about the best first.

I love to flirt.

Flirting isn't just for romance and sex, flirting is for everyone. Babies flirt with us in restaurants. Dogs flirt when they want us to throw a ball. Hummingbirds flirt with the very air. I flirt every time I notice some fun, beautiful, connecting energy and I decide to notice it and play with it.

What is flirting? How can we spot it? How can we get really good at it? Why would we want to?

I have two images of what it is like to flirt. First, I envision flirting as playing together with energy like tossing a Kush Ball back and forth, like kicking around the hacky sack, like soaring a Frisbee across a freshly cut lawn, like shooting squirt guns on a hot summer night. There is a lot of laughter, smiling, rising to the occasion, and double daring each other to be creative and cute and clever, bringing out the best in us.

It doesn't matter if it is in-person or through an adorable text or within a Facebook poke because when we flirt we are really saying *I like you, I am thinking about you, you're awesome, let's play.*

The second image I have of flirting is surfing, catching the massively fun energy of a wave and riding it. You see it coming and you start paddling and you join the energy of the wave. You don't try to control the wave, you just ride it. If you love surfing, there are and will always be waves to catch because every minute of every day there are millions of waves building behind millions of waves peaking behind millions of waves high-fiving the shore. There are always flirting waves of energy to catch and enjoy because the desire to connect playfully is always deep within all of us.

As fun as flirting is, it has always gotten some bad press. Flirters are frequently judged by others. Why? It seems that flirting sparks jealousy because when we flirt our energy goes from spreading out far and wide to everyone and everything near us (remember the electricity balls from Chapter 4?) to a laser beam focused on one or a very few others. And if that beam isn't on us we feel left out.

So sometimes the people who feel left out judge the people who are flirting. They say things like, "She's such a flirt" or "He's a player" or worse they just say whatever will hurt us. This happens so often that flirting is almost considered a negative thing, as if flirty people are just a moment away from being sluts or players.

Not true. Flirting is great. Flirting is simply playing with our energy. Just playing.

Try not to judge others who are flirting. Just notice that you feel left out when others are flirting. Try to remember how great it feels when you are flirting. Don't hurt the flirters. Be happy for them. Join them if you can. On the flip side, when you are flirting, try to include more people. Notice if anyone is feeling left out. It's easy to include others. Get good at flirting.

How?

First, remember we are all born knowing how to flirt. Because flirting is usually paired with sexuality and is often judged in a crappy, moralistic way, we sometimes forget how to flirt. But like riding a bike, once you become aware of how it feels, you will always be able to flirt when you want to.

The easiest way to catch that flirt wave is to look for the best in the other. When we do this, they usually look for the best in us. Our protective force fields can come down and then we can play. It's hard to play anything when you are carrying a huge shield. That's why babies and dogs are so good at flirting. They have no shields. We have no need of shields when people are seeing the best in us. The best way for people to see the best in us is to see the best in others. Super simple.

Flirting. Do it. Do it often. Notice when someone is inviting a flirt. Their eyes meet yours and they smile. They text something funny. They shove you playfully with their shoulder. They notice you. They tease you. Then watch how you respond to them, how you relax and enjoy and tease back and play. Try and do that with others. The easiest way is to see what you like in the other. That's like showing a dog a ball. That's all it takes.

Gripping the moment kills it. Don't start thinking about buying the person you are flirting with some BFF necklace. Don't start marrying the girl or guy in your mind as you toss the ball back. When the energy of the moment begins to lose its momentum, be grateful for the moment then then get your board and head back into the ocean to catch the next wave.

I hear you saying, *What the heck Molly, flirting* is *about sex not Frisbees and surfboards.* Not so, but the best romances do begin with a flirt. My brother Jo Sha interviewed a guy who said his favorite kiss ever was the one during which he and the girl smiled through it (see Chapter 21). The best romances do begin during a flirt. If there is a flirt and a hint of romance or sexuality, then, my friend, you are on first base.

Because flirting actually creates more energy than the energy that started with each person (two plus two somehow equals ten), flirting is the best way to start a relationship. Great romance needs a lot of energy. Flirting provides it. I leave a flirting moment all filled up: happy, smiling, and deeply knowing my worth. In what better soil can a romance grow?

I say we change the definition of flirting to being aware of the beauty and divine worth and fun in someone, and acknowledging the awesomeness directly through smiles and laughter and play.

Flirting is all about loving the life in others, laughing, being present right here, right now. We can flirt away a whole lot of problems like hatred, loneliness, and self-doubt. We can flirt our way into some great romance and smiling kisses. Like the Hokey-Pokey: *That's what it's all about!*

TWELVE

virginity is not a backpack

What an odd thing virginity is. One minute you're a virgin, the next you aren't. One simple action. Does that go for the other orifices? Are you a virgin nose picker until you first put your finger up your nose? Do you have virgin ears until you use a Q-Tip? I don't know.

Having sex is this amazingly personal thing—what you put and where—yet with our generation we talk about it like we talk about our backpacks. You have it. You lose it. Your friends want you to lose it or keep it. It's a burden. It defines you.

In reality, it is an experience, not a possession. Almost everyone I've talked with said the actual moment of "losing it" was such a letdown compared to what everyone thought it would be. When I was younger, I thought the moment I lost my virginity my life would change from Dorothy's black-and-white Kansas into the brilliant-colored Land of Oz.

To be honest, that is what happened when I had my first orgasm with Joe, and that wasn't sex. I was still a virgin after that. For a long while, colors were brighter and the world more magical.

In the book *Memoirs of a Geisha,* there is a huge commotion over which man will be able to pay the highest bid to have sex with the geisha first, to de-virginize her. This goes on for months. The entire time the girl is terrified, but preparing herself. Finally, this one guy pays a ton of money. The girl waits in this room lying down on a mat. The guy comes in, gets on top of her, penetrates her, moves around a bit, and comes in an instant. Once he is done he collects a little of the fluid mixed with blood that comes out of her, like some souvenir, and leaves. She never sees him again.

The best part of the whole thing is after he leaves she is sitting there with the masterful geisha and the two begin laughing at how ridiculous the whole thing was—how much drama, money, and preparation for such a shallow and unsatisfying and silly event.

More than likely the first few times boys have sex they are going to come very fast and girls are going to hurt. The movie *American Pie* and the book *Anatomy of a Boyfriend* describe first-time sex between couples who had been together for awhile and who had been on the other bases quite a few times before.

The first time probably won't be the best thing that will happen in your life and hopefully it won't be the worst. It just is. Certainly you can do lots to make sure it's a good experience. You can choose your partner wisely. You can make sure you are safe. You can make sure you are really ready. You can study sexuality. You can know your body. You can make sure you have already mastered self-pleasure and orgasm. You can have skill in talking to your partner about sex. You can make sure you aren't harming your belief system.

And, truly, if you've had sex and chose to stop having sex for a while in order to practice, to learn, to master, then you can still be virginal. Especially if that first sexual encounter was bad or forced

Try not to make your first sexual experience one that will produce guilt, shame, embarrassment, fear, anger, disappointment, trauma, or drama. These have nothing to do with sexuality as an art form. Why have sex if these will be the result?

Quick Note. I know this book makes it seem that I am against abstinence. I'm not. I am against *abstinence-only* sex education. I actually believe abstinence is certainly one alternative. Especially now. I think it's better to wait and learn and practice than have sex with uninformed, porn-trained high-school boys. (Let's face it, *abstinence-only* is geared way more to girls than guys.) It's a great way to say *no*—you can twirl your abstinence ring or say you are waiting until marriage. It's a great way to ease your parents' fears while you are waiting. They'll let you out of the house and let you text way more if you tell them you are waiting. It gives you breathing room. It can connect you to your family's beliefs. It can be a holy pause.

I hate the *only* part. I hate it because it says you have to wait until marriage, (which we've established only about seven percent of the population does) and it gives no alternatives. It teaches *abstain or ruin your body and become a slut* and that simply is not true. If it were true, then 93% of all adults would be sluts.

We can choose to abstain. I believe we can also change our minds when we are ready, and we can still be healthy, safe, loving, and beloved by God. Otherwise, heaven is one empty place and hell is as packed as Walmart on Black Friday.

THIRTEEN

exercise in self-pleasure

I can't believe I'm writing this, but really, someone has to talk about it! This is the part where we get specific about not letting anyone else teach you about your body but yourself. Besides, too many girls aren't having orgasms. Too many boys just self-pleasure mindlessly. This is a recipe for sexual disaster. So here goes.

Here's an exercise for conscious self-pleasure. (For God's sake, make sure you're in some private place!) Notice the emphasis on focus, on building excitement, on slowing down and not just racing to the orgasm. Notice your entire body.

Think about something sexy: someone who turns you on, some great chest or abs, someone's flirty eyes or smile, some scene from a movie that stirs your body.

Think of it.

Now, without touching yourself (no matter what's going on down there), focus on your circuitry. Feel the firing of electrical impulses from your groin to the rest of your body. Feel this. Notice your mind wanting to go further into the imagined sexual act. Note your hands aching to touch yourself.

Don't.

Not yet.

Relax.

Notice.

Quiet your mind for a few minutes.

Now, think that sexy thought again. Touch yourself.

If you've self-pleasured before you already know what feels good.

If you haven't, take your time.

There is a lot to explore.

Find spots that thrill you, that heighten the tingling everywhere.

Then stop.

Move your hands to the rest of your body. Lightly caress every inch of yourself. Note the circuitry firing like tiny electrical shocks. Find which areas feel great.

Remember, take your time. Stop and start. Relax. Begin again. Notice your whole body. Notice your thoughts. What images or fantasies are flashing at you?

Go slow.

Build. Build. Build.

Discover your sexual body.

Make it come alive.

Find its pleasure.

At some point you'll pick up the pace. Your body will tense up. Even though your focus will be on your groin, notice the rest of your body and mind.

Do what feels great.

Build and build.

Before you release, be ready to notice the big bang throughout your entire body. Notice the pure peace and ecstasy and connectedness.

When you're there, release.

Oh...my...God!

Yep.

Oh...my...God...

Feel your heart rate. Feel the blood coursing through your body. Feel the electricity flowing fast and pure and unblocked throughout your system. Feel the enormous pleasure of the release.

Know truths you often forget—especially that you are not separate from anyone, from nature or from God. Know your infinite worth.

Practice. This is where your sexual energy needs to go first.

Know thyself.

Don't let some other teen try and teach you about yourself.

We might decide to wait to have sex, but we can certainly enjoy the pleasure of our bodies while we wait and learn and master this sacred art.

If you have a hard time having an orgasm with this exercise, there are some more specific ideas and exercises in *Our Bodies, Ourselves*. In Daria Snadowski's book *Anatomy of a Boyfriend*, the main character, Dominique, never experiences an orgasm with her boyfriend, even though they've already been having sex. Her best friend gives her a vibrator. There is a great section about her finally having an orgasm using the vibrator. It's worth a look.

FOURTEEN

porn

First and foremost, you don't need it. You don't need anything to get turned on. You're turned on all the time. Old guys in boxer shorts sitting alone in a hotel room need it. Couples who have been married a million years and barely like each other need it.

Porn is to sexuality as cancer is to health, as junk food is to fit bodies, as greed is to the soul. But...Let's face it...Most teens have seen porn, just like most of us have eaten junk food now and then. So let's figure out how to deal with it.

Porn today is not porn of yesterday. It is not photos of naked girls with big boobs or guys with tux ties and thongs.

Hard core porn today is accessible, private, and dangerous to your sex life.

Here's why. You're sitting around, horny. You're curious, you're human. You have access to the Internet, which is private and lets you look at anything you want, parental controls or not. Without adults giving you wisdom about sex, you use porn as your classroom. Porn isn't real sex, and it misleads you in two ways.

First, porn sex occurs about thirty seconds after the first badly acted "Hello." You begin to believe that sex is a moment of attraction and then a quick devour, like eating a burger in your car when you're starving. You skip most of first base, all of second, all of third, and just get it done.

I think we've already established that bodies don't naturally just go from a hello or a kiss to being ready for sex. We don't work that way, especially female bodies. Yet in porn, the women are always ready for anything, anytime, anywhere, with anyone and everyone.

I hate to be sexist, but it does seem that girls understand that porn is fantasy way more than boys do. I hear girls say time and time again that they think porn is stupid because "those girls are not having any fun" and "they are so faking it." Those girls are right. There are books full of horror stories about what happens to the porn actresses: how sexually abused they are, how they have to be drugged up to have the things done to their bodies that are done while filming porn, and how physically damaged they are by this. I don't understand why girls see this and boys don't.

And yet, many still believe that normal girls are always sexy and ready for sex. We aren't. Porn is a fantasy. It's as real as Peter Pan's flight and Harry Potter's wand. Say it with me, "Porn is fantasy. Our bodies don't work that way."

Good sex is not super quick with someone you don't know at all. It isn't degrading. Good sex doesn't include actions that harm women's bodies. Porn does.

The second reason porn is dangerous to your sex life is that you look at some fairly soft porn. You start to get pretty excited, and, whether you ask for it or not, the porn hardens. It gets more wild, violent, twisted, but—and this is important—you're really turned on. So stuff you wouldn't usually think about, you begin to think about. You begin pairing being turned on with images that will alter your thoughts, fantasies, and desires. Images of kids or animals or violent sex can begin to turn you on. It's hard to have a great sex life if these images or things turn you on.

Whereas mindful sex is about connecting with the other, porn is about disconnecting. Mindfulness is about equality and respect. Porn is about dominance and disrespect. Mindfulness is about healing. Much porn is about exploiting, abusing, and injuring.

And remember, you're really turned on. Your sex life will never be the same because you begin to like fast, disconnected, demeaning, disrespectful, and injurious sex. This won't stay just in your horny teenage years. It will be in your thoughts as you become sexual with someone you really like—your girlfriend, your boyfriend, your spouse. You'll be at high risk for porn addiction. You'll be at high risk for high-risk sex. You'll be at high risk for failed relationships.

It's all about the energy. Porn is about taking energy. Mindful sex is about blending, sharing, and creating energy.

If you want to look at healthy sexual images, go to your local bookstore. Most have sections of books on sex and erotic literature. They aren't considered porn. They're just books on sex. There are drawings and photos of people having great sex. I go all the time and get a cup of chai and do my research. Who knew there were so many ways to have sex? I get plenty turned on by these books. Anyone can buy them. They'll turn you on and teach you about sex without ruining your computer or your mind.

The other day I went to a bookstore and sitting on the ground right by the *Sex and Intimacy* section were two teenage girls looking at these sex books. They weren't embarrassed. They were having fun.

Like with fast food, a lot of you are going to ingest porn. So, like with fast food, try and keep it to a minimum. And don't believe it is good for you, and don't believe it is real. Okay?

FIFTEEN

cyber-sexual connection

We're the first generation to be able to get sexual online. It's easy. It seems safe. You can say and do and try things you'd never say or do or try in person or even over the phone.

People see your profile on something like Facebook. You put a sexy picture on it. You say if you're a virgin or not. You make some sexy name or song or answer to a question.

And you get offers, lots of them. And just like I mentioned in the chapters on bases, some of these offers go from "Hey, wassup?" to some pretty sexual encounters. Except they're only in words. Sometimes it's a game. Sometimes it's a way to get turned on, have some fantasy you can self-pleasure to.

Because there is no accountability like in real-life interactions, harmful things can occur. Be mindful of them. Let me give you three examples.

First, boys these days, even some really great boys, try to collect naked photos of girls like they used to collect Pokémon cards. They ask, and girls almost always tell them *No*. But they keep asking. They are relentless. Girls often give in and send them a photo, and these boys often send these photos to all the other boys they know. It is so disappointing. It hurts so many girls.

I have a favorite cure for this, ladies. Every time a boy texts you and asks for a naked photo, forward that text message to every girl you know. More than likely those boys are asking lots of girls for nude pictures. Then all the girls can shun that boy and embarrass him, the way the boy sending your photos around to all his friends would embarrass you.

Right now the boys have the power when they beg and beg and then send your photo to everyone. Take back that power by forwarding their requests and warning all your friends. That should change things up. And *never* send a nude photo!

Second, you can't know if you truly like someone you've only met online. It's body to body, eye to eye that tells you. Some great flirt online might do nothing for you in person. One of my older friends met up with this guy she met online who she was sure she was going to marry. He flew a long way so they could meet. She was so disappointed by the flesh and blood guy who showed up. Even though he did indeed look like his picture, he just didn't excite her at all. Sex is all about flesh and blood.

Third, there are the stories of old and dangerous men posing as cute, sexy boys trying to get girls to have cyber-sex with them or meet with them. Gross! But how can you know?

If someone starts getting way more sexual than you feel comfortable with, BLOCK THEM. Blocking is a great thing. There will still be a million people contacting you, just get rid of the Bozos.

Basic safety rule: don't give your address or school or work or any information that could lead someone you don't know to you. If you decide to meet, meet in public and make sure you have a friend nearby if you want to bail. Do not go meet someone alone, ever. If you meet them, and trust them, then treat the relationship like you would any other relationship you met in real life. Otherwise, wave them good-bye, and block them forever, and if they are way older than they said, report them.

You have all these opportunities. Make sure they are what you want. Make sure they are what you want published because this stuff is public for the rest of your life, including for future bosses and lovers and even your kids.

SIXTEEN

connect and disconnect

There is a belief in Zen Buddhism that most people we encounter in our lives will come and go rather quickly. There will be a very few that last forever: family members, some best friends, husbands, wives, children.

Most people will come and go. This is natural. If we kept everyone forever we'd be overwhelmed with the time and energy all those relationships would take.

Most relationships are moments. Good or bad, they end.

For some reason when we really enjoy a moment with another person, we have this need to make it last forever. We go from enjoying and seeing the best in the other to clinging, to expecting more than the moment.

Then, when the relationship either naturally ends or is choked to death prematurely, we decide we must feel terrible about it. We weep. We get angry. We decide that the person was never the great person we thought they were. We decide they lied or manipulated. We discount the moment we had. We doubt ourselves.

This happens times ten if attraction, romance, sexuality, and especially if sex occurred during the relationship.

Let's face it, all sexual moments do not end in marriage. In fact, only one or two will.

Don't hold on to relationships. Assume they will end some-time. Enjoy them. Don't pretend this cute boy won't move on in ten minutes or two days or three weeks or six months. When you know this you'll make informed sexual decisions.

I hate to say this, but ladies, I see so many of us acting like we're going to marry every random guy who flirts with us. I hear girls crying because they had sex with a well-known player who said "I love you" before the first kiss then disappeared after the sexuality or sex. Your bad. Really. If you know a guy is a player and is going to move on quickly, then decide if he's someone you want to be sexual with. Simple as that.

Be honest. Because most relationships are short, don't do things you only want to do with a really long-term relationship unless it's been really long term. Don't get all hurt when the flavor of the week moves on.

I also hate when people get so mad they get vengeful at their exes. They act like these very nice moments they had were completely fake. They act like the guy or girl was really horrible when in reality most of those moments were real and nice and sacred. Yet just because they didn't end in a long-term relationship the experience is made pathological. What a waste of great moments. When we could have these great mental scrapbooks of great moments we rip them to shreds instead. How messed up is that?

I have a friend who makes the boys she goes out with promise they will have a Mutual Breakup. They promise they won't lie to each other about their feelings. She thinks we all know when a breakup is inevitable. There is a magical shift and nothing—no kindness, no great sex, no gifts, no meanness, no threats, nothing—is going to repair it. So she and the guy promise when that happens they admit it and breakup at the same time. So far it's worked nicely.

Why don't we just admit when it's over? Do we really want to stay with someone forever when it is gone, when the connection is broken?

Let's be the generation that quits being all hurt when relationships end. Let's quit being vengeful. Let's quit cursing those souls we loved for a blessed moment or two.

SEVENTEEN

safe sex

Sexuality is a tricky thing. Though I hate all sex education that begins, ends, and discusses only the safety aspects of sex, a sexual master must know the risks and precautions.

Sex is risky because we're emotionally and physically vulnerable. Like with any risky experience, you have to be prepared. You don't skydive without instruction and certainly not without a parachute. You don't have sex without being safe, without protection, without responsibility.

The obvious physical risks are pressure to go further than you want to go, sexual assault, pregnancy, and sexually transmitted diseases (STDs).

Pressure and Sexual Assault. I was surprised when Jo Sha told me a lot of the guys he talked to felt like they went further sexually than they felt comfortable. Some felt the girls skipped most of first and second base and were rounding third, heading for home, way before the guy was ready. If the guy tried to slow down, the situation rumors quickly spread that he was gay.

Girls reported time and time again they were simply kissing a boy when suddenly their pants were off and they felt they had no choice but to have sex. Or even though they were not giving any signs they wanted to go further, the boys were going fast and the girls had a very hard time saying "No."

We should know the signs that our partners don't want to go further. The signs are obvious, so there are no good reasons to ignore them. (We went over these in detail in Chapter 9, *Third Base*.) The main sign is that your partner isn't going forward. There is no heavy breathing, no body pressing against yours, no pelvic grinding into you. The other isn't leading your hands places on their body. They aren't taking off pieces of their own clothing for you to explore.

Ask the question "Is this all right?" Or "Do you want to..." Only an enthusiastic "Yes" is a true yes. No answer is a "No." An uninspired "Okay" or "I guess" is a "No!" and certainly a "No" is a "No" is a "No!" no matter what you've been doing up to that point.

Sexual assault is just a step further than going further than you want to go. Usually it involves someone not listening to you and forcing you to go further than you want. Ladies, I know we think we're invincible, but guys are stronger. Simple as that. If you are alone with some guy who decides to force sex, you will probably lose any battle you put up. The safety basics are the same for pressure and for sexual assault.

Safety Basics. Know what you want and what you don't. Never be so alone with someone that you can't get away from them.

Don't be sexual in a house with no one else there if you don't want to have sex. Blame your overprotective parents even if your parents aren't overprotective and don't have a clue where you are.

Don't go to parties or camping in the mountains or the desert or anywhere out in nature if you don't have your own car and if you don't know the people well.

Don't go to any parties alone where you don't know the people well. As with hiking or scuba diving, always have a buddy or two with you who won't leave you.

Never go into a bedroom with someone you don't know.

Don't get drunk or high and sexual.

Don't talk about sex or have cyber sex with someone you don't know then meet up with them alone.

Have a bunch of ways to say "No" or "I don't want to do this" way before you start down any of the bases.

Finally, talk with your potential partners. Ask them what they want to do sexually. What have they done before? Not everyone will be honest. I hope you can tell the difference. I hope you take enough time to find out about them before you become sexual. Either way, if you talk to them they will know your line. Then you can draw it if the situation goes too far. You'll have a better chance of using your voice if you've set up the situation first.

Pregnancy. No kid wants to get pregnant. Not one teen Jo Sha or I interviewed wanted to get pregnant. I've heard about girls who want to get pregnant to trap their boyfriends or get out of school or bad home situations, but I don't think that happens as much as it did in the past.

Potential pregnancy is the number one reason teens don't have sex. We all know we wouldn't be the kind of parents we hope to be. We wouldn't be financially ready. We wouldn't be in the right relationship to parent.

So be responsible. We are baby-making machines right now. Please remember this.

Jo Sha began asking boys who had sex with a lot of girls about condom use. He said a bunch of them refused to wear condoms. He began asking these guys about their partners.

"So, dude, all these girls would make great mothers for your kids, right?"

"You want to be part of all these girls' lives forever?"

"These girls will make great babies?"

I guess they all went running to the store for condoms!

Don't get pregnant. You don't have to. First, really, don't have unprotected sex unless you don't mind getting pregnant or having an abortion or adopting out a kid.

No one should be without birth control if they are being sexual. All cities and most towns have some sort of public health center that gives out free condoms and birth control. They are almost always staffed by kind adults who want to help us not get pregnant.

It's really hard to take yourself to a place like that for most teens. Kids drag their feet even though they know they are at risk for pregnancy. Get your best friend to go with you. Or better yet, go with your partner. Or get some adult you trust. It's easier to go if you can go with someone.

We have a perfect chance now to never have unwanted pregnancies. We're the first generation to have this. There is now a pill we can take within a few days after unprotected sex that will not allow our bodies to get pregnant. It isn't the best way to not get pregnant, but if you make a mistake you don't have to get pregnant. You can get these at the Health Department and over-the-counter at the pharmacy.

Sexually Transmitted Diseases. STDs are no fun. Some of them are mildly annoying and mostly can be gotten rid of by taking medication. Some are life-long horrors like the herpes virus that leave you with canker sores you can spread to your partners. Some are deadly like HIV.

That's why being sexually intimate must be something you do consciously. Random partners are dangerous because you don't know what they might transfer to you via semen, lubrication, and blood. At that cellular level you are having sex with everyone they've had sex with.

Condoms help a lot. But mostly, you want to be with clean people who have respected the hell out of their bodies.

If you slip up and have sex with someone you don't know or trust, go get checked at the health department. It's usually free or affordable. Make sure you are safe and healthy. Don't spread anything. It is just wrong.

Here I'm giving this huge lecture on safe sex, yet I know it is easy to be unsafe. I know the night I was with Joe I would have had unprotected sex if Joe hadn't stopped it.

This is important.

I knew him well. I'm pretty sure he hadn't had sex before. I'm pretty sure he wasn't a player telling me he was a virgin. So my body was probably safe from assault and STDs, but certainly not from pregnancy.

Still, I was so swept up in the moment, in my desire. I had no clue I could ever feel that turned on. Now that I know how great I can feel, I never ever get into sexual situations without taking care of my safety.

EIGHTEEN

sexual abuse

About one in five of us have been sexually abused in one form or another. Someone did something sexual to us that we didn't want.

Sexal abuse can range from children who are perpetrated on by adults to teens seduced by people in positions of power to make-out sessions that go further than one of the parties wanted. The acts can range from being spied on, to being fondled, to oral sex, to penetration in any form. These can be subtle or blatant, seductive or violent. The perpetrator can be a friend or stranger or a relative.

Regardless, the experience can mess up your sex life if you don't heal from it.

It can make you afraid of all sexuality. It can make you ashamed. It can make you disrespectful of your body and your sexuality. It can spark flashbacks as you become sexual. It can arouse in you sexual feelings you didn't want to have.

That's the bad news.

The good news is you can heal. The experience lasted hours or minutes of your entire life. It doesn't have to mess up you and your sex life forever. Millions of people have healed up from sex abuse to have perfectly fine sex lives.

First and foremost, you have to make sure it isn't a secret. Tell someone. Tell everyone. Let it out. Release it. The power the perpetrator tried to take from you is in the secret. Within the secret is the guilt, shame, fear, blame, and self-hatred.

Tell someone and get help.

Most teens are afraid to tell anyone about the abuse because they are afraid no one will believe them, or that the perpetrator will hurt them, or someone they love will go to jail, or worse, they will lose control again. Remember, you have all the control now—it is your body, your memory, your desire to heal and/or stop the perpetrator.

Your future sexual happiness depends on you getting help from who you want, in your time, in your way.

NINETEEN

just stop

Stop.

Stop using sexual words to injure others. Really, we have to stop.

No more....

Slut.

Whore.

Fag.

Pussy.

Fucker.

Cunt.

Dick.

Lesbo.

Ho.

We are so much better than this.

These are the same damned words our parents used...and their parents used. Do you want your sex lives to be like your parents? Then stop making sexual words the same words you curse others with.

I know it is fun and powerful to swear. It makes you older. But, really, all these words pair someone you are angry with to sexuality. Sexuality becomes paired with negative things.

We hurt our sexuality to call some cowardly kid a *pussy*. A pussy is not a horrible thing. It isn't a weak thing.

I know this sounds stupid, but it's not.

Stop calling bullies *dicks*. What do you really want to say to them? *Back off? You're a jerk? I hate what you did? You scare me?* Otherwise you're saying a dick is a bad thing. If you believe dicks are bad things and pussies are weak things, our future sex lives suck.

I mean isn't "Fuck you" an offer?

We call girls we're mad at *whores* and *sluts*. We call girls who flirt with guys *whores* and *sluts*. This implies that every girl who pisses us off sleeps with lots of random guys. We're saying all sexuality makes you a prostitute. It has to stop.

Worse than all this is calling each other *homo, fags, lesbos, gay* when we're angry at each other. To me, this is worse because we're absolutely saying being gay is bad. It's really cruel and wrong. It took this country forever to stop using racial slurs like *nigger* and *spic* and *chink*, but somehow it's still okay to use *gay* and *homo* as slurs. Even gay kids use them.

No matter how much you try and say that using these words doesn't hurt our sex lives, you know you're wrong. You know the power of words. You know how words like *stupid, lazy, fat, ugly, loser* have hurt all of us. We just can't use our powerful, glorious sexual body parts and actions as swear words. We just can't.

In his book *The Four Agreements*, Louis Ruiz challenges us to be impeccable with our words. He swears if we work hard to say only what we precisely mean, then most of our problems will vanish. He believes this is an easy way to happiness and peace. So how can we still be powerful and cool and express our anger and fear without cursing our sexuality? How can we be impeccable with our words?

I mean I guess we still have *bitch, asshole, shit, bastard,* and *damn* when we need to swear. Maybe we can make some others up. I know a woman from Italy who screams *Porka Miseria* and shakes her fist when she's mad. It's pretty fun to use. I think it means *misery of the pig,* though I wonder if I'm missing something in the translation.

I wish we had much, much better skills in dealing with conflict. I know we can do better. We can stop hurling sex words at each other every time we feel hurt or incompetent or furious or jealous or sad. We can make it totally lame to curse others with that list of words. Don't let anyone get away with them. If you need some acceptable curse words, make some up.

TWENTY

change the rules, ladies

Some boys are going to want to become sexual masters. They're going to learn to be great partners. They'll know to flirt and hold hands and kiss softly. They'll know the bases and take their sweet time. They'll enjoy getting to know you. They'll realize how amazing it is to connect with you. Some boys are going to become great lovers in their lifetime.

Reward these guys. Wait for them. Insist upon these boys for friends and boyfriends and lovers and partners, like the boyfriend in *Juno,* Nick in *Nick & Norah's Infinite Playlist,* the great boy in *Adventureland* and *Zombie-land.* Make these the popular boys.

Please stop rewarding the old model of the sexy beast. Stop voting the predatory, stupid, cruel boys as Homecoming kings and guys everyone wants to date. Stop. That's all it takes. Cruel boys need to be shunned sexually and socially. They need to be ignored. They need to not get reinforced.

Why is this cruel boy still the model for popularity? This is the same model our mothers and grandmothers used.

These boys are mean. They steal our power. Yet we give them our attention, attraction, and bodies. Stop.

We are no longer Neanderthal chicks who need the strongest guys to hunt for our meat. We are quite capable of taking ourselves to The Bell for our burritos. We no longer live in a society where only big, strong, stupid, and aggressive men can support us and our future families.

These guys scare us. They thrill us. The cross all sexual lines. They go from, "Hey, wassup?" to "Are you a virgin?" to "Give me a hand job."

They are notoriously bad at sex. Really. They don't even know this. They only know they want quick and frequent release. Do not be the vessel for some jerk's quick release. He has a hand for that.

Begin insisting on great guys. Guys who are friends. Guys you can talk to. Guys who are kind. Watch them around animals and children and adults. Those jerk boys might call the good guys *pussies,* but really, *pussies* are rather fabulous things. What's wrong with a boy who's as great as a *pussy*? Call them what you will, I say they're fantastic.

Insist upon the very best for you and your body. Is the boy a jerk or great?

How many girls has he had sex with? (This information is usually readily available.)

How many girls has he hurt?

How quick did he go from "Hi" to sexual talk and requests?

How kind is he to others?

How confused and pressured do you feel?

How much do think you can change him? (The more you focus on how much he'll change if he's with you, the bigger the jerk he really is.)

Does he know anything about sex as a sacred art?

A lot of boys are great but have no clue about the bases and the sacred arts, so teach them. Ladies, it is mostly up to us to make this change happen. We can change the world one boy at a time.

TWENTY-ONE

dudes, alter
by Jo Sha Top

Molly asked me to write this part. Unlike her, I'm not gonna talk about my sex life. I did interview a lot of guys, and I think they had some important things to say.

First, let me talk about something that's not going to change. Let's get real; most of the time all we want to do is insert. Yeah, all the time. *(You can substitute 'insert' for a thousand different words. I just didn't know what could be published!)*

Our bodies, our young bodies, are all about inserting. We were made by God to insert.

So how does any of this stuff Molly's saying make any sense to us? Cuz there's no great art form to inserting. My dog, Spud, he's trying to insert all the time. He's working other dogs, our couch, my leg. No doubt, there's nothing sacred about old Spud's want for inserting.

So if the goal for most of us in inserting and coming, who cares about connecting and energy and holding hands and violins and all this B.S. Molly's writing here?

We do. I swear. When I asked these guys, they said they actually care. I mean inserting was their primary goal, but they wanted to know the sex was good for the girl. They wanted to be with a girl they liked. They wanted to feel good. They wanted the girl to feel good.

I like the way this one dude described a good relationship: *I liked this girl a lot. She was so cool. She was comfortable with her body, her hot body. We laughed all the time. It was awesome because when we kissed, we smiled. Yeah, I wanted to fuck, but I really liked her, too. We waited a long time, and we actually never did have sex. We did, like, everything but. It was way better than the actual sex I've had.*

When I'd first start an interview, the guys would say, "Yeah, I've had lots of sex." Then when we kept talking they told me some stuff, like a lot of dudes feel kind of weird right after they have sex. They wonder if the girl feels bad about it. They wonder if they went too far. They really wonder if the girl came too. They all wonder about the girl coming.

They also felt weird after sex because sometimes the girls got all clinging and all I love you-ish. They felt obliged to go out with the girl, but they already felt weird about not knowing if they were any good at sex and if the girl came and all that. It just seemed like a lot of them felt awkward after being really sexual.

I know guys are afraid that people will say they are gay if they don't have sex with as many girls as possible. You aren't. What a crappy reason to have sex.

I say, "Be choosey." Just because you can have sex doesn't mean you have to have it. My hand and a little lotion have saved me from a lot of Chainsaw Massacre kinds of scary relationships and their eventual breakups.

TWENTY-TWO

let's do it

I've said it before—it's time for a revolution, a sacred sexual revolution.

When I think of revolutions, I think of riots and anarchy and anger and flipped middle fingers. Yet the most successful revolutions come more from intense commitment of a large group of people to do something different from the well-established rules of society.

Let's recap why we need a sexual revolution. Here are the sexual rules we live with:

We are told to abstain from sex until we marry in our mid-twenties.

We have access to pornography and cyber-sexuality from a very young age.

We live in a culture that bombards us with sex, mostly to sell things.

We have bodies screaming for sexuality from about fifteen years of age.

Ninety percent of our swear words pair anger and hatred with sexual body parts and acts.

A lot of us have been sexually abused.

We have zero education on healthy, creative, playful, connecting sex.

We are minimally supervised by the adults who make and enforce these rules.

Many generations back have lived by these rules.

To do it differently, we have to know our power. We have to commit to ourselves, our sex lives, our future partners, and our kids' sex lives. We just have to.

Change is hard. That's the revolution...change. We have to do so much differently than our parents, than our peers. We need to do this together. We need to demand a lot from each other.

Change the sex terms. Change the cuss words. Change our views on self-pleasure. Stay away from porn. Explore sacred sex texts. Be mindful. Demand sexually mindful partners. Heal up from sex abuse. Go slow. Learn and practice.

Let's become sexual masters.

Let's save the world through great connection.

THE END

ABOUT THE AUTHOR

Molly Top is forever nineteen and bellybuttonless. She was born as a character in a book by Elizabeth L. Clark when an amazing boy named Joe needed a perfect girlfriend. Whereas Joe stayed in the book, Molly jumped from the bindings and wrote a book about great sex lives.

If you want to know what she looks like, look in the mirror. Her voice is yours and that of every other teen who's had questions, fears, experiences, desires, and hopes for their sex lives—their right-now and future sex lives.

The difference is that while you all sat through Algebra and took out the trash and stood in the endless photo line at prom, Molly Top forced Elizabeth to interview a zillion people (or slightly less), study about ancient cultures' attitudes and mastery of sex, and write a book for you, for us...so we can all have great sex lives.

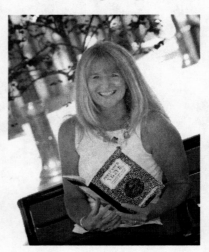

Besides channeling Molly Top, Elizabeth L. Clark loves riding her bike downhill.

Find out more at MollyTop.com.

YOUR OWN NOTES

CPSIA information can be obtained at www.ICGtesting.com
Printed in the USA
LVOW052219070912

297716LV00004B/2/P